Quiet Highways

Quiet Highways

An Empowering 3-Step Journey for Parents of Autistic Children

Britt Olizarowicz

Text copyright © 2020 by Britt Olizarowicz
All rights reserved, including the right of reproduction in
whole or in part in any form.

Do you get to choose?

I chose the quiet highways
I chose museums on Mondays
I chose the mid-week vacations
I chose the restaurants at 3:30
I chose nonfiction over fiction
I chose knowledge over sleep
I chose the truth
I chose to give up on fashion and accept clothing
I chose to count a granola bar as dinner
I chose homeschool
I chose therapy for all of us
I chose love
I chose to adjust
I chose to learn
I chose to comfort
I chose routine
I chose calm
I chose home
I chose patience
I chose to lose a bit of control
I chose to not lose too much control
I chose to help as best I know how

When you asked me if I got to choose if you were born with this,
the answer is no. But I would choose you a million times over.

With all my heart, autism or no autism, I choose you.

CONTENTS

INTRODUCTION 1

Three Stages of Mental Health Care in Parents
of Autistic Children 7

FIRST STEP:
APPROVAL

Understanding	11
Dealing with Diagnosis	27
How to Handle Blame	33
Key Reminders from the Approval Process	41

SECOND STEP:
ACCLIMATION

Letting Life Change	45
Expectations and Goals	59
Communication	69
Eliminating Comparisons	73
Key Reminders from the Acclimation Process	81

THIRD STEP:
AMPLITUDE

Fuel for the Bad Days	85

They Just Don't Get It	91
Empathy and People	101
Key Reminders from the Amplitude Process	105

AFTERWORD
Remembering Your Role — 107

ADDITIONAL RESOURCES — 111

ACKNOWLEDGMENTS — 113

ABOUT THE AUTHOR — 115

Quiet Highways

INTRODUCTION

THINKING BACK to my childhood, I always felt as though Mom knew exactly what to do. At all times and in all situations, she knew what was right and what was wrong. She knew what was good and bad; she knew who broke the plate even if nobody fessed up to it. Sure, she was overwhelmed at times, but overall, she knew how to parent. She was my mom and *that's what moms do.*

I never even thought about or wondered *how* she knew what she was doing—at least not when I was a child.

I never questioned where she got her knowledge. As a young child, I didn't even question if there were other ways to do things. If Mom said that's how it was done than that's how it was done.

When I was pregnant with my firstborn, I spent countless hours worrying about how *I* would know what to do. My mother seemed to possess hundreds of years of training, like she was born to be a mother. Surely, I would have to learn this in some other way. It couldn't possibly come as naturally to me.

Google searches, blogs, and parenting books seemed like the only logical solution. How else could I get all of these answers and ideas that my mother appeared magically born with? Being the oldest of three children, babysitting for thousands of hours, and completing a degree in elementary education, I had spent the better part of my life with and around children. I had some general idea of how they function. Still, I questioned, did I know those rights and wrongs and good and bad like she did? Did I have enough knowledge to make this whole motherhood thing work out?

Ready or not, March 3, 2014 was the day I became a mother. That was the day it all made sense to me.

After a terrible pregnancy and an emergency induction I held my perfect baby. Looking at him and holding him for the first time it felt like I had known him for a million years and we were just meeting up again.

That's when it hit me.

My mother didn't actually have all the answers.

All those years growing up, when I thought she knew it all, she questioned herself. I realized she stayed up late worrying about whether or not to let us have juice boxes. She lost precious moments with us by saying, "Be careful" or "Not too fast." She criticized herself as a mother and knew at times that she made mistakes. She tried to make beautiful memories for us when it came to holidays, celebrations, and birthdays, and sometimes it just didn't work out. From the eyes of a young child, none of this could be seen. Only through the eyes of a New Mother did I realize she too was fallible. She never really had all those answers. And neither did I.

All we have is instinct and love. That's it. The rest is a big ol' Google search/mom group/family advice/self-help book/gamble. The two constants—the things you can continually return to—are instinct and love.

My mother has good instincts and she loves me to a fault.

The definition of a parent is rather simple. All you have to do is have offspring. Any grown adult knows that this dictionary definition needs about an eight hundred-page edit. Parents come in all shapes and sizes, just as children do. If you are reading this book, you likely have upped your parenting portfolio to that of "Special Needs Parent" or "ASD Parent." Those badges expand the parent definition well over that eight hundred-page mark.

When I first realized I was heading down the path of becoming a Special Needs Mom, I didn't see it coming. I was still so busy trying to figure out the whole parenting thing. I had been at it for only about two years, and in the grand scheme of things that's not a very long time. I didn't pay enough attention to the "Special Needs" aspect creeping up on me. Now I try to think back to what it was like without the autism glasses on and I almost can't remember it.

I do remember worrying about the future of my child, but not in the same way. I remember worrying about the independence of my child, but not like today. I remember worrying about little meaningless things, like Easter outfits that matched and the perfect wipe dispenser. Now things like that never cross my mind.

I compare it to learning to read. Remember when you would constantly have to ask, "What does this say?" Everything seemed interesting, new, and positive. Once

3

you learn to read, there is no going back. You can't look at a stop sign and unread what it says. You just read it. Same thing with ASD parenting. Once you put those glasses on, they don't come off. Your world will never be viewed in the same way.

I've been in this game for several years now and come to realize that there is a true difference between parenting and parenting a child with ASD. The same rules and regulations do not apply. The same roles and responsibilities do not fit.

Is it harder? We will get to that.

Is it more demanding? Yes, without a doubt.

Is it more rewarding? We will get to that as well.

My motivation for putting this all down on paper is a very meaningful one. For a long time, I tried to convince myself that I was just like any other mom. My kids still need to be loved, to eat, to sleep, and to play. This, of course, is all very true. I can relate to other moms; I can see that all kids go through some of the same things in life.

The problem was, by trying to pretend that everything was fine and that I was just like any other mom, I unknowingly put a great deal of pressure on myself. My everyday mindset was, *It could be so much worse*. I was trying so hard to stay "normal" that I was making things much harder than they needed to be. The pressure to conform to the social norms of today's world was unrealistic and unattainable.

The straw that broke the camel's back was when I saw a blog post about "Self-care for Moms." I read the post because I knew my "self-care" was lacking. Spa days and nail appointments just don't fit in. I struggle with time away from my children and many times it's not worth the hassle. While I was reading the post it hit me that since this autism thing changed our world, I have come a long way with my *mental* self-care.

If your everyday mindset is working and you are managing and enjoying life, without desperately needing spa days and independent trips to Mexico, then maybe you are on to something? Truthfully, I had no other choice than to get myself to a healthy and meaningful mental state, so that I could function as the person my children need me to be.

I have changed who I am and how I think. I've learned how to "care" for myself in a way I never thought I would. I needed to understand and work through what was happening to my family, my life, our world. The process I went through, the journey I have been on, should be shared. If I can save just one other parent from the time, the pressure, and the heartache that I put myself through then putting this all on paper will have been well worth the effort. Keep in mind as you read on, I'm a mother to a child with high-functioning autism. I only know *our* story. I don't have all the answers. But I live every day on a journey to find solutions to make the future of my family the best it can possibly be. There will be things that differ from you and the journey you are on, but I know in essential ways our paths as parents are very much alike.

THREE STAGES OF MENTAL HEALTH CARE IN PARENTS OF AUTISTIC CHILDREN

PARENTS OF autistic children are some of the most stressed and sleep-deprived people in our community. This type of parenting takes being a caregiver to a completely different level. Not only do you have concerns about your child and their physical and mental well-being, but there are many other factors. Parents of autistic children are dealing with social stress from the outside world by trying to conform to social norms. They are dealing with financial stress because of therapy and diagnosis and treatment, in addition to missed work days to take your child to these appointments. Thinking about the future of your child and all the work, effort, time, and money it will take to get them to be independent is enough mental stress to take down even the strongest people in our society.

At some point in this journey I recognized that I had developed an effective way of handling the weight of being a parent to a child on the spectrum. I have no problem admitting to the fact that being a parent to a child on the spectrum can feel like a weight. It sort of drives in, drops itself off, and doesn't go away. For me, it was just a way of life. I walked around carrying the weight while trying to live the same life I always did. This doesn't work. After a series of experiences, both good and bad, I was led to a new mindset. I decided to work backward to break down how I got here and what it took. After months of thinking about this and analyzing, I concluded that there are three main parts to parental life on this spectrum.

Although many parents are not going to be able to take the physical break that they all might need at times, these mindsets and mental workouts will ultimately positively affect your mental health. They can be implemented at home today; they are simple and easy to remember and will change the way you view the world you are in. If you can plan that spa day or that trip to Mexico, by all means go for it. But if you are like me and that just isn't in the cards at the moment, please try these steps. Both you and your child will benefit greatly.

The three steps in my system are: **Approval**, **Acclimation**, and **Amplitude**. By the end of this guide you will be able to determine where you are in this process, how to complete each step, and be able to start looking at your life through a brand-new and very clear set of autism glasses.

FIRST STEP

APPROVAL

(OF YOUR CHILD, OF YOUR SITUATION,
OF YOUR LIFE, AND OF AUTISM)

10

I.

UNDERSTANDING

If you were asked if you enjoy golf or tennis better, you may have an opinion. But if you never tried either sport it would be impossible for you to choose which one you like more. Let's take this a step further and say that you are only allowed to play golf. You have no option to play tennis. Of course, you might wonder about tennis, and at times fantasize it may be better than golf. It may even bother you and seem unfair that you can't play tennis. Eventually you would have to approve of golf and learn to like it. It's your only option and you only get to live once. If you chose *not* to enjoy golf, you would miss out on all its enjoyment.

Even though you would eventually learn to love the game of golf, there would be quite a bit to learn. But since it is your only option for a sport, you might as well be good at it. It's going to take a great deal of time and practice to educate yourself. It will take hard work. It will take research and diligence. There will be times that you think you should give up and times that you think you may finally have it all figured out. This process can be both enjoyable and rewarding if it is approached from the correct mindset.

OK, let's reframe the metaphor.

When you became a parent, you most likely did not get to choose ASD parenting. (Some cases of adoption might prove otherwise.) As shown in my simple golf/tennis example above, since ASD parenting is your only option, it needs to be approved of. The more time spent wondering *why* this has happened to you will only postpone your destination of peace, happiness, and understanding. Why the neighbors' kids are "just fine," and you are sitting there with a kid in just underwear working on the same puzzle for the fourth time that day, will do you and your child no good.

The fact that you can't go to that Mommy and Me class because you are in therapy with your child is hard to approve of but it needs to happen.

Not being able to send a Christmas card because your child can't tolerate family photos (why does this always have to be a thing?) is difficult but it's not going anywhere.

The sooner you can approve of this process, this lifestyle, and your child, the sooner you can make progress toward your goals, and more importantly, your child's goals. And the easier your life will get.

So how do you go about this approval process?

Understanding in this situation is a two-part process. The first part is understanding what autism is. The second part is understanding how your child is affected.

You can't properly approve of something that you don't fully understand. Doing so would be an uneducated misstep. When I first learned about sensory processing disorder (how my son's high-functioning autism first appeared), I was extremely confused by the terminology and the actual concept. The sensory system is a very complicated part of our body. A loud noise presented to him early in the morning could lead to him not eating well later in the day or a meltdown two days later—unless on the same day as the loud noise we did some rock climbing, trampoline jumps, or scooter boarding.

At first, when I learned about this process of seeking and non-seeking and proprioceptive and vestibular, my head spun (something I was used to watching my son do numerous times a day). For instance, my son would be melting down, but if I asked him to pick up a weighted medicine ball and carry it across the house, he would "recover" and regulate himself.

There were days when I felt as though I was on *Candid Camera*, that this couldn't be real life. It couldn't be real that if I wanted him to tolerate walking into a shopping store, we would have to swing for twenty minutes prior. Then even after doing all the swinging and planning and prepping we may still have to walk out should we encounter an unexpected occurrence (like the music being louder than normal). I was so caught up in the steps of how to *handle* this process that I didn't focus on what sensory processing disorder (and eventually autism) were. Not just knowing the medical terminology but truly understanding how it works and affects the body.

Understanding your child's diagnosis—what it is and how it affects them—is the only way to continue to progress and move forward. It takes time to read and learn about autism. Find blogs, Facebook groups, or Instagram accounts that can help you and your child. Look for local support groups. Try to make one friend with a child on the spectrum. Ask your child's therapists tons of questions. They may seem as though they are the expert—and when it comes to their field, they are—but when it comes to your child, YOU are the expert. You are their full-time therapist.

Reading a definition on Google is not going to cut it. You will see a broad description with a bunch of keywords like "social issues," "communication issues," and "fixed interests." This doesn't help, as these are all symptoms, but they don't explain *what* autism is and what your child's autism will look like. It's going to take quite a bit more time, research, and work to understand the complexities, the cause and effect, and most importantly, the depth that is involved with this condition.

One thing that helped me from the start is the realization that we were all in this together. My son doesn't go to therapy; WE go to therapy. It's a team effort.

He's never sat through a session alone. His sister, his father, and I have all gone to therapy with him. I've never caught up on Facebook in the waiting room of a therapy session. Sure, at times I've had to sit outside so that he can work on some things independently, but I listened, I learned, I questioned, and I researched.

Going to therapy is not something a child can do on their own. It's kind of like telling a child to potty train themselves, or handing them a bike and saying, "Ride it." It just doesn't work like that. That is why WE go to therapy.

All the therapists we have met through the years have become great friends and amazing resources. They know I'm going to come in with questions; they know I'm going to come up with things that we need to work on. They know I listen and watch every single thing they do. They know my goals will be lofty. But most importantly, they know that *I* know my child is capable and I care about him and the progress we are making.

The therapists have not only taught me but inspired me to learn more and to do more. Watching therapy sessions helped me understand both autism and the way autism affects my child. Had I not been able to witness these sessions there is no possible way I could have made the improvements and adjustments in our home that have led to so much progress.

For example, when my son was almost three, I had to stop at a bank to make a deposit one afternoon on the way home from occupational therapy. When we pulled into the bank's parking lot he said, "This is a different bank." I told him that it was just closer to the therapist's office but it was the same Bank of America like the one he is used to. This was before I developed the superhuman power of anticipating 97 percent of meltdowns. I never saw this one coming.

We got out of the car and he was talking faster, very anxious, worried about walking into a "new" bank. As we got closer to the door, I realized his legs were completely locked up and before I knew it, he was lying on the pavement, screaming. He said he couldn't go in.

15

People came in and out of the bank, most of them leaving us alone. An older woman stopped and said, "He's not a very good listener." It took everything in me not to give *her* something to listen to, but I let it go and focused on my son. I talked him down. We did some breathing. We pointed out how similar this bank was—the layout, the color etc. Eventually he decided he could handle walking in. When I got to the counter, they said that I required one additional piece of paperwork to make the deposit I needed to that day.

I cried.

The bank teller had no idea what had happened. I knew he thought I was nuts, but I deserved to cry after that. We left the bank and I explained to my son that I couldn't get done what I needed to and that we would have to try later that afternoon. Immediately, he said, "That's fine, but we will go back to our old bank." Every ounce of me, every single part of who I am and who I want to be as a mother, wanted to say, "Of course we are going to our regular bank; I would never attempt that again!" The thing is, we had just come from therapy. Had I not just sat in on the session about not letting your ASD child control your entire life, I may have just caved.

Instead, because of my UNDERSTANDING of autism and how it affects my child, we went home, got the paperwork, and went back to that same bank. This time he walked in without any trouble. He even told the bank teller that he planned on being a doctor someday. When we got back to the car he said, "It's not my favorite bank but I can handle it."

At our next therapy session, I told the occupational therapist the story. She was busy working with my son and I was just kind of talking in the background about what I did and that I hoped it was right etc. She looked up, made direct eye contact with me, and said, "You are an OT now." Of all the things I think I've ever been called in my life, this one made me the proudest.

Had I just read that definition on Google, had I made the decision to leave autism to the experts, we would have lost this learning opportunity. And it was an important one.

What therapists have learned about me is that when I go home, the changes are implemented. Their work, the time they put in with my child, is honored and respected and it is carried over into our home so that we can make a real change in our lives and the life of our child on the spectrum. You should be saddened when you walk into a therapy office and see signs about making sure your child shows up for therapy, or asking you to be sure you are back by the time their session is complete. Don't let your child feel like they are in therapy alone. Tell them WE go to therapy.

When my son started behavioral therapy, for the first few months I got way more benefit out of it than he did. He would even ask me if we were going for him or me. Always, my response is, "WE all go. WE all need it."

Currently, we homeschool our child The combination of giftedness, anxiety, SPD, and ASD was enough to make us realize that traditional school at the moment is not the best fit. I have no complaints about homeschool and I think it is one of the best decisions we have ever made for our child. I kept thinking about where he would fit in the classroom. I just couldn't picture the right fit for him and I honestly didn't think it was the school's responsibility to find this fit. Education is a system. It's created to educate mass amounts of people. It's a good system, but it just doesn't work for my child at the moment.

In the same way I didn't expect the school to find a place for my child, I don't expect a therapist to single-handedly impact or change the life of my child. It's my job, my responsibility, and my calling to help him. That is why WE go to therapy, so that we can understand autism and understand him.

Start to own the fact that at the end of the day you need to know more about autism than any other person. Don't expect other people to become the expert. Be the expert your child needs you to be.

Only when you understand the entire scope of the condition can you start to comprehend the impact it has on your child. Without true understanding, some things that are autism related are just going to seem behavioral and vice versa. I know that as my knowledge grew, there were people (mostly family) that thought I was nuts when I would say certain things were related to my son's sensory system. I'm sure I sounded ridiculous but I was right.

I was right that he couldn't handle preschool.

I was right that we shouldn't be forcing him to eat new foods.

I was right to tell him everything in our upcoming week, month, and year.

I was right to tell him the truth that shots hurt and that medicine doesn't always taste good.

I knew that his lack of sleep was not because I wasn't being tough enough on him.

I was right that not all parts of the holidays and celebrations need to happen in the traditional matter.

These were not simple parenting instincts. I questioned myself just as heavily as I was questioned. I had to *research* to know what was right in this situation and for my child. I had to increase my UNDERSTANDING so my child would suffer less.

Were mistakes made? Absolutely, and they are still made every single day. The point is that I understand autism as well as his occupational therapist does. I know how to explain how autism affects my son to his behavioral therapist. His pediatrician and I don't need to discuss autism in detail because he knows that I know more about how it affects our world than he ever could.

I can now not only help my child but also another young mother in the community who is still in those days of head-spinning madness when food is being thrown at you and your child won't put clothes on. It's not the terrible twos. It's not a "threenager." It's autism and it needs to be understood, researched, and learned before moving forward.

Once you have a decent understanding of what autism is, you need to understand EXACTLY how it affects your child. Being that this is a large spectrum that we are working with, this condition will not be the same in your house as it is in mine. The most difficult things for my autistic child may come easy to yours. Meeting other parents of autistic children can help you feel like there are similarities between your family and others but no two stories are ever the same.

When learning to understand your child there are several things you can do to help speed up the process. During the day, mentally record some positive and negative moments. When you have a few minutes to yourself at the end of the day, go back through those moments and learn. Why did the meltdown happen? What happened thirty minutes prior that could have triggered it? Family pictures, a new pillow on the couch, blueberries. . . how would that cause a meltdown? Look in your ASD Moms Facebook group. I near-guarantee someone talks about how and why each of these things has been a problem for them too at some point in their lives.

It's important to make mental notes of the positives as well. What made your child happy today? When did they seem relaxed, well adjusted, and less anxious? What caused those things to happen? Start to build your life plan by these little moments. The process seems extensive, and it is, but it is the only choice to eventually create peace in your home and help your child thrive.

It took me years to feel like I had the full scope of how my child was affected. We had to experience many new things together to figure out what was going to cause issues and what wasn't. Travel, play dates, school, seasons, family events, weather, sibling issues, holidays, illness, etc. There is still so much more we have yet to experience and

I have no doubt that autism will impact these things as well. As we were all taught in school to "learn from history," you need to use your prior experience to prep and plan for the future. Don't put too much pressure on yourself to figure this all out in a weekend. You won't.

The holiday season immediately following when my son was diagnosed with sensory processing disorder was terrible for us. We brought down all of our boxes of decorations eager to show him. We let him pick out the tree and decorate it. We played Christmas music, changed our routine, and headed to all the "fun" family events for children in the area. It was all a disaster. I remember being so concerned about him having memories and holiday traditions, I wasn't focusing on the triggers. To me, the holidays have always been such a happy and exciting time. I never even thought that it could possibly throw him off.

What I have come to learn about the holiday season is that it is a very intense, overwhelming, and sometimes unnecessary marketing scheme. We have completely changed how we do Christmas at our home and every year since has become so much more enjoyable. Now we understand that moving furniture to put up a tree is actually incredibly stressful for him. We prep, we plan, we move less, and we keep the tree up for a short period of time. One year we even asked him if we should skip the tree. He didn't want that.

Each year we have learned about other surprising triggers. For instance, going to Home Depot during the holidays. They are usually playing holiday music overhead yet they also have holiday decorations that play competing music at the same time. This is like a sensory explosion and it's terrible, so now we stay out of Home Depot. Too many gifts on Christmas morning is also a problem. The smell of Christmas trees, candy canes, and holiday-scented candles—all a problem. Too many people, parties, outside distractions—it's *all* a problem. Before I understood autism and how it affects my child, I would have never thought of any of these things being an issue.

Our holidays get simpler each year yet the memories are better. As my son gets older, he can communicate more about what triggers him and what doesn't. Just this past year he told us that glass Christmas decorations put on mantels make his head hurt. He said cluttered things like that just don't look good and are pointless. My husband and I looked at each other and realized he was absolutely right. We were putting out decorations that had been passed down to us through the years for no other reason than that they had been passed down. Our son doesn't live like that. If it doesn't work for him, it doesn't happen.

Paying attention to your child's world will help you have a better understanding and ultimately a better chance to aid them when the difficult situations present themselves.

When you get your official diagnosis, they will likely give your child a level of autism. The levels have been created to help better define the autistic spectrum. Before these levels, there were five different diagnoses that were considered part of the autistic spectrum. Unfortunately, these diagnoses were confusing. Different practitioners selected different diagnoses for the same patients. In fairness, at the time there was truly no easy way to diagnosis autism. To clarify their diagnoses, practitioners (as well as teachers and therapists) used terms like "severe autism," "mild autism," and "high-functioning autism." These terms, however, aren't true diagnoses at all; they're just descriptions of autism. And while they were intended to help parents and teachers better understand a child's status on the autism spectrum, each practitioner had their idea of what "mild" or "severe" might look like.

This became extremely frustrating for parents and children alike.

Today, your child will be classified as level 1, level 2, or level 3. Knowing this information will do nothing to help you with your next steps. It simply puts your child in a category. Sure, you can look up a list of best practices but you are going to have to dive quite a bit deeper to find out exactly what this means for you, your child, and your family.

Oddly enough, a child who is level 2 autistic might function better than a level 1 at times. This can happen when triggers are not being managed or therapy is not working etc. Maybe the level 2 child is extremely regulated while swimming and functions much higher than the level 1. As you can see, these levels don't mean anything. It gives you a starting point but truly does nothing when it comes to UNDERSTANDING how this affects your child.

This process of learning what your new life will be and what autism even is will take time. I remember looking at moms of autistic kids who were a few years older than mine and thinking, *They must be true experts.* I had no choice but to become the same thing for my child. When the diagnosis happens, you feel like a freshman in high school (or maybe a kindergartener)—everything is new. Therapists and family and physicians are telling you what to do, and you're not even sure how or why this is happening.

Take it one day at a time but try and learn. My son couldn't fall asleep unless I laid beside him each night. I ended up making a deal that I would lay with him but I had to read something on my phone. As he drifted off, I looked at mom groups and mom blogs and articles about autism. I studied it like it was my major in college. It came easy. The information was not hard to remember because I was applying it in my everyday life to help my child.

My level of understanding my son has gone up and down through the years. There are times when I know thirty minutes before a meltdown it will happen because he made some simple little face and I combine that with the fact that there was thunder last night. Other times I'll say something as simple as "Let's play on the swings" and it causes a meltdown. I don't quite have everything figured out but I understand him and his behavior better than I've ever understood another human in my life. I've learned to be a better mom and I've learned that by understanding him and autism it gives me confidence as a mother. The worst possible thing for a young mother to feel is that she has no idea what she is doing. It leads to a bad self-image and mental state and it needs to be avoided at all costs. Don't let this happen to you. Read, watch, observe, and study. This is your life and it's here to stay. In the long run, you will not regret a single minute you spent learning how to understand your child.

2.
DEALING WITH DIAGNOSIS

Just like autism is a spectrum, no ASD diagnosis is the same. Some are diagnosed very young; others are diagnosed when they are twelve or even thirty years old. I do believe from my own experience, and other parents I talked to, that by the time you get the diagnosis you know it is coming.

We noticed signs of sensory issues right at the two-year mark, but we were dealing with very noticeable advanced speech and IQ. Closer to two and a half, the behaviors were no longer "neurotypical" and it was obvious to us and many around us. We started occupational therapy and were told it was sensory processing disorder almost immediately. We didn't get the autism diagnosis until five years and one month. I can't say during that period that I was truly seeking a diagnosis, but I wasn't avoiding it either. In my heart, I'm pretty sure I've known since the first day he toe-walked across our house.

Between the time we started occupational therapy and the time we got our autism diagnosis, I wasn't bringing him in for evaluations to get a true answer. We were working on life making more sense for all of us. We were working on keeping some sense of normalcy. We were trying to preserve and maintain as much of that early childhood happiness as we could.

When earning my elementary education degree, any chance I got to take an elective was often about exceptional children. The signs, the red flags, the quirky behaviors—I knew what to look for and when, although at the time I couldn't believe they were appearing in my child. The diagnosis came as meltdowns were getting worse and more behaviors were emerging. The difference between his cognitive age and emotional age were getting too wide to hide it anymore. The high IQ part helped to push our diagnosis off a few years but it was always there.

The diagnosis process is a process to say the very least. The evaluations are time-consuming and meetings with the psychologist can be exhausting. For me, it was a mental struggle that lasted for months. I fell into a bit of a hole, gained about fifteen pounds, and just sort of felt lost. Our road, although difficult for years, had almost seemed like it might turn away from the autism diagnosis. He made so much progress early on in OT (and my tolerance and understanding had grown) that a small piece of me held onto the idea that maybe it wasn't autism.

But it was and it is.

The question is, *It's the life we have been living for years, so why did the diagnosis hit me so hard?*

That small chance that it may not be autism was gone. On the good days I sometimes liked to pretend things might be normal. On the bad days, I held onto the fact that it might just be a bad day. All that was gone.

I felt sorry for my son, for myself, for my husband, and my daughter. This went on for a few months. I remembered the joy of telling my husband I was pregnant,

28

and getting to share with him it was a boy. Those moments are some of the best of my life. They strengthened our marriage and made us the family that we are. Having to then tell him that I thought we needed our son evaluated, and that It was SPD, to eventually come home from the psychologist and having to tell him it was in fact autism—it's not a day you think about when you picture parenthood. It's not an easy thing for a marriage to handle. It's an experience where you feel as though you are an outsider in your own life just trying to manage all that is coming at you. It's loss of control.

One of the most challenging things for me in dealing with the diagnosis process is that everything else around you is still going on. You are trying to focus on the fact that your child might be autistic while also taking care of them, their sibling, the house, the business, the dinner, and the list goes on. It felt sort of like carrying thirty buckets of water and being told not to spill a drop.

Then there is the marriage aspect. I handle the fact that our son is autistic in a much different way than my husband does. My patience level is naturally higher than his because I'm around the kids more often. He tends to be more productive than I am at heading toward a solution. I give my son more time, letting things try to happen naturally.

We handled the diagnosis differently. When a father is told their son has autism it affects them in a way that they have a hard time explaining and verbalizing. There is sadness, guilt, blame, hope, amazement, curiosity, fear, and about thirty other emotions tied together. After dealing with a day of work, the house, the bills, and the kids, we are supposed to sit down and discuss *how we feel* and how this massive freight train that is taking over our lives is affecting us? It just doesn't happen—at least not effectively and it becomes increasingly difficult. We struggled not to talk about it too much that we ended up not talking about it enough.

Communication is such a key factor in any relationship and when the outside world causes so much pressure that communication lacks, the real problems start to arise.

All the things I had dealt with for years in this sensory/autism world, the diagnosis was the hardest for me. Looking back I wish I hadn't let it impact me the way that it did but I have learned from it. I worried a great deal about having to tell friends and family and hearing the different responses.

I did not want to hear "Oh, I'm so sorry."

I also didn't want to hear "He's fine, he will be fine."

I honestly have no idea what I *did* want to hear. All I know is that nothing anybody said felt right and having to tell people that your child is autistic also doesn't feel right. At first.

I'm very careful to say that my son is both autistic and gifted. I once described him as "so brilliant BUT he has autism." I was upset at myself for thinking of it this way and from that day forward made a very conscious effort to never say "but" he has autism. There are plenty of advocates who will stand up and tell you that autism is a wonderful thing and it shouldn't be looked at negatively.

30

I don't negatively look at my son at all. I never will. I do however look at autism in a negative way when I see the way it makes his life more difficult.

There is no doubt his life is made more difficult by autism and in turn, there is no denying that my life has been made more difficult. Not better, not worse, just filled with many moving parts. This is why the diagnosis becomes such a huge part of the approval process. When it comes to receiving this news, it is black and white. You have no choice but to approve of the diagnosis and move forward towards acclimation. You can believe your child is the most amazing, high-functioning, brilliant, beautiful person in the world. I sure do. He is also autistic.

Without approval of the diagnosis, you cannot move toward helping your child in the way they need. So how do you approve a diagnosis you never wanted?

Productivity.

Feeling sorry for myself and our family didn't last very long. The truth is it can't last very long. There is a task at hand and you need to roll up your sleeves, put on your big kid pants and start dealing with the reality of what your life is. This part is not difficult. There is a ton of research out there. The people in your community will help. You will have a certain amount of natural instinct that will guide you as a parent. This is the part when you get to show your child how much they mean to you. You will be able to share stories with them about the pretend play beach trips you had together where you learned how to potentially have sand touch their foot. When they get older you can tell them about how you would call museums to make sure they didn't have a field trip that day or see if they would maybe let you in just twenty minutes early. On top of parent and caregiver and just about everything else, you become your child's greatest advocate. This task can be quite rewarding at times.

The single most important fact about approval and diagnosis is that your child has not changed. Your world just changed. The future changed. What the neighbors think has absolutely and permanently changed. But your *child* has not. That can be a difficult feeling to separate and hash out but it's extremely important to remember you are dealing with the same little person you dealt with yesterday, even if you now have a diagnosis.

3.

HOW TO HANDLE BLAME

A natural feeling when it comes to the step of approval is blame. This situation, your life, your child's struggles. . . Why? Who did it? What happened? These are all normal feelings and nothing you should be ashamed of. Blame is defined as assigning responsibility for a fault or wrong. It only seems natural that if something is considered "not right" with your child that you would look for a cause.

Through the years many people have asked me about vaccines, family history, genetics, and environmental factors. It's not just the parents of the child that want to know—all people want to blame somebody or something for autism.

Blame is simply a way to try and have this all make sense. If someone or something is to blame then that is the reason it happened. Without that blame, autism just sort of floats around ready to land in anyone's house, at any time, and it makes it scary and unfair. The average person wants to take steps and measures to keep autism away from their child. Many of us (autism parents) say that we wouldn't change a single thing about our children, myself included. If, however, their lives were simply made easier from the start, if autism had never happened, I would have gladly accepted that.

When I first started seeing signs that my son had sensory issues, I didn't want to believe it. For a month or so I tried to write it off as normal toddler behavior. Then I went through the stage of thinking it was just me knowing more than I should know about toddler development and I was "looking" for problems. And then I went through the stage of blaming myself. It was an ugly time and it completely consumed all of my thoughts and emotions. I felt as though I couldn't relate to family or friends, and sometimes my husband. The burden I carried was way too much and something I wish I never did.

One of my goals in sharing our story is that other parents do not put themselves through what I did. When blaming myself started, it looked something like this.

SLEEP

I figured that even though I read all the books and articles about proper bedtime routines and sleeping patterns, I must have messed it up. We tried cry it out, don't let him cry, bath at night, bath in the morning, books, no books, swaddled, not swaddled, sound machine, no sound machine. Sometimes something would work for a day and we thought we had it fixed, only to find out it truly lasted for a day.

The lack of sleep starts to affect your brain as a parent and you truly begin worrying about your child's ability to learn and function and grow with the small amount of sleep they are getting. So even though I spent a long time researching this, questioning friends and convincing myself that I had "messed up" his natural sleeping patterns in some way, I was wrong. As hard as I tried to take all the blame for this, it's not me—it's autism. My son just can't get his brain to settle enough to sleep through a night. He is on sensory overload by the end of his day, regardless of what occurred. He has slept through the night four times in his entire life! I've adjusted to it at this point and even therapists and psychologists have said, "It's just an autism thing." It felt good to release this from my list of potential parenting faults.

I stopped reading articles about sleep in children; they just don't apply. I donated the children's sleep books and I just gave myself the APPROVAL that this was not my doing.

EATING HABITS

My next round of blame started with the eating habits. I had determined that he was a picky eater because I didn't expose him to enough great food. The reality is that I made all of his baby food by hand. The kid never had anything from a jar, or processed, or not homemade for almost two years of his life. This is still funny to me, as I now smile with pride when he eats a Ritz cracker, willingly.

I put so much time and research into making baby food and planning meals and introducing new food. I just thought that wasn't enough. I thought because my husband and I have a pretty traditional diet that I ended up making him picky. When he liked a food, I would give him more of it. I had myself convinced that must have been a mistake. When he was down to about three to four

35

foods and we started occupational therapy, I learned that NONE of this was on me. There are things about food and texture and smell and taste that I never knew. All of these things impact his sensory system differently. When I thought my son was being picky and giving me a hard time, it was not because he wanted to. It was because he literally could not try a new food.

Eating new foods is still a major battle for us. It can take a month to add one new food, only to have it drop from the diet one day with little to no explanation. I still beat myself up when I grocery shop and debate how I'm going to piece together nutritious meals for him for the week. The lesson here is that now I have APPROVED of his diet. It is what it is. I constantly work to help him grow and try new foods, and he works just as hard at it. I can't blame myself for his eating habits. It has nothing to do with me and everything to do with autism.

ROUTINES

My next area of self-torture was the routine problem. Sure, you hear it over and over again that children like routines. It's good for them. They *want* structure. Well, I happen to like routines myself and I believe in a routine that is planned out and accommodating to children. I had my babies on schedules very early on and overall it worked great for us. In my opinion, there is no need to fill a child's schedule without any regard for naps and meals. All of those things need to come first. But when my son

COULD NOT stray from his routine, I started blaming myself for getting him on one to begin with.

He struggled very much with being able to transition from one activity to the next, especially if it was unplanned. When we were playing a game and would decide to go outside it almost always resulted in a complete meltdown. He loved going outside. In fact, he loved being outside more than he loved being inside, but he still couldn't break the routine. What I eventually came to learn is that this is a control thing. If his day goes according to routine, he's great with it. If he's playing with something, and it's time to transition to the next activity, he struggles because he was content and in control during the first activity. It was a safe zone and he is worried about what the next activity will be like for him to process.

As hard as I had originally tried to blame my boring and organized self on this love of structure and control, it wasn't because of me. Autism, yet again.

CLEANLINESS

I presumed he didn't like to get dirty because he was my firstborn and we constantly made sure he was clean and neat and ready for a photo-op at any time. I let him try finger painting and sand play and messy chocolate cake. All it did was upset him. So, I blamed myself. I thought I wiped him up too much, worried I changed his diaper and his clothes too often. I saw other moms saying to their kids "you are fine" and I had a change of clothes for mine.

It had to be my fault. I must be the reason that he couldn't go to a beach or a park that had sand.

Now after years of occupational therapy and increased knowledge and understanding I have learned that his sensory system just doesn't process things the way they should. Sometimes he does things that help him regulate and he becomes a seeker, and other times he is a complete avoider. What I do know now is that none of this is caused by me making him wear shoes in the yard or not letting him walk around with food all over his shirt. It's just him and how he works.

DIFFICULT PREGNANCY

The worst one for me has been the pregnancy. I question every day of that pregnancy. I question the gestational diabetes. I question the pre-eclampsia. I question having to be induced a day before thirty-seven weeks. Each and every time (and there have been many times) I've had to fill out an evaluation and they ask the ever-popular duo of "Difficult Pregnancy Y/N" and "Born before Full Term Y/N," it rips me apart. It was out of my hands, not something I chose. But I went right to the guilt the day we were told it was sensory processing and again the day we were told it was autism. I stayed there for several weeks completely convinced it had to be from me before I realized that this was ridiculous and ineffective. *Nobody knows what causes autism.* Someday we may know, and that might take away this blame card, or it might put it right back on me. For now, the reality is that this is not helpful for my mental health. Parents of autistic children are in a difficult mental place to begin with; casting of unnecessary blame is only going to further stress the parent.

What has helped me deal with all the negative self-blame? What has helped me to APPROVE of myself and what I have done to help my child? It's a simple solution and one that you can implement today.

Blame yourself for the GOOD things.

I'm the one who recognized his behaviors were not age-appropriate or neurotypical. I'm the one who made that difficult call to the pediatrician and said the words, "something isn't right." I'm the one who sat through every single OT session, went home and implemented the strategies, changed my life, our life, our home, my plans, my career, my everything to help him. I'm the one who stays up all night when he needs it. I'm the one who knows what triggers him and how to back him down when he gets into a bad place. I'm the one who is there on the good days *and* the bad days. I know how to defend him, how to protect him, and how to encourage his independence all at the same time.

All of these things I deserve to blame myself for. All of these things I had control over and I will take full responsibility. Helping your child succeed is the only choice you have. Parents of special needs children tend to focus on the negative in their lives. They expect a great deal and put a tremendous amount of pressure on themselves to make life better for their child. It feels like you have no choice and that is a heavy burden to carry. The gap, the missing piece is that special needs parents don't get the credit they deserve for the good things. It's rare to get compliments and praise for the job you are doing. And although it is a labor of love, there are days that it can feel like a job. One with no overtime, no sick days, and no retirement!

When your child sits through a dentist's appointment, it wasn't an accident. It's because of how you prepped and planned and worked for it. It's the time that has been put in therapy and social cues and reading about it and talking about it. None of this is an accident, and the letting go of blame is an imperative step in the approval process.

The next time an idea comes into your head about something you may have done (or your spouse may have done) to cause autism, it needs to be immediately dismissed. How are you going to master the step of approval and fully welcome the fact that this is your life, your story, if you are still trying to figure out who or what caused it? You won't find that answer. Even if you could find that answer right now, you may not like it. Let it be. Let go of the blame and learn to approve and accept the fact that this is here to stay. Put those autism glasses on and wear them proud.

KEY REMINDERS
FROM THE APPROVAL PROCESS

- First, you need to understand what autism is and then understand how it affects your child.

- Make sure to attend and participate in therapy sessions. Each one is an opportunity for you to help your child.

- Diagnosis is supposed to feel difficult. The emotions and struggles are all normal and need to be dealt with.

- Blame does you and your child no good. Only blame yourself for the GOOD things.

- Approve of this life, approve of the future, approve of everything because it is not going anywhere.

- This is not a process that anybody is going to do for you. It needs to be done by the parent and every minute you put in will be worth it.

- Nobody knows what causes autism.

42

SECOND STEP

ACCLIMATION

(RECOGNIZING AND EMBRACING THAT THIS IS
GOING TO CHANGE EVERYTHING)

44

1.
LETTING LIFE CHANGE

When I look back to the early years, right after we realized there was a problem, this is what I see:

- A very pregnant (with her second baby) thirty-year-old mom who thought she knew what was coming.
- A mom who thought more OT appts a week = more progress.
- A mom who thought, *Thank goodness it isn't "really bad."*
- A mom who googled way too much.
- A mom who tried to control almost every aspect of our lives to keep things "safe."
- A mom who tried to explain this all to friends and family but never felt like she was understood.
- A mom who focused way more on the latest and greatest sensory bin or swing than she did on her own mental health.

If I could go back, there is one thing I would say to this mom. It's the one thing that could make things easier, take the pressure off, and make her feel so much less like a failure. I would say, "Stop pretending that this doesn't change everything and just let it."

Just let it change everything.

The most obvious first question is, Why?

Why let this unexpected neurological condition come in and change my entire world? My child's world. Our plans for the future and our idea of parenting and life with children. Why let it change the way I keep my house, how we travel, our marriage, what we do during a week, schooling, eating, and so on. You name it—it has changed.

Because it's going to anyway.

There is not a single thing in our lives that is left unaffected by our child's diagnosis of autism. Not all of this change is bad. Not all of this change is good. But the point—and you need to understand this from the start—is *it's going to change everything.* The more you fight this, the harder it will be on you and your child.

How you react to this change and "acclimate" will define both the success of you and your child.

If you are new to this, the idea of everything changing may seem scary and overwhelming. You need to trust me on this and learn from my mistakes. Trying *not* to change is a much worse alternative.

MY HOME

My couch was once a place to sit down after a long day. Now it is sort of a trampoline/sensory gym/upside-down hanging chair. It has been used to make crash pads more than it has been used to sit on and watch a movie. All our furniture is utilized for sensory integration, fort building, and occupational therapy. We bought a trampoline to dissuade jumping on the bed. It helped a little but not enough. His room is closer to ours than our baby's room because he comes in multiple times a night and needs to know we are close. He first climbed out of his crib when he was fifteen months old. When he was young, we had extra hooks and locks on the outside doors.

Things at home are organized. Every single thing has a place. If it moves from that place, it can cause distress. The rooms are orderly. We don't own fancy things. If we change a piece of furniture or a pillow or a rug, we can expect there to be an issue, a complaint, or a meltdown.

This is fine; we have accepted it. If it takes a bit more organization and a little rearranging to make our home safe and sensory-friendly, we are all for it. We let him pick his room color (within reason) so that it felt like a safe zone for him. He was three and promptly chose black. We settled on navy. The home changes have had the least effect on me. I love a nice clean, neat, well-decorated home. I'm still able to do this and have it be a nurturing and positive environment for my autistic child.

MY MARRIAGE

I was recently speaking with an engaged woman who mentioned that the pre-marriage lessons offered by the church were very helpful in preparing individuals for any issues that could come up in a marriage. This comment had me laughing. If you are religious or not, there is nothing that can prepare you for marriage with a special needs child. No church figure can explain to you what you will feel, what your spouse will feel, and how that will impact your marriage. It's not possible. For those who are religious, the church can be a great support system but it can't prepare you for what you have coming. The only way to know how this will affect your marriage is to see how it affects your marriage.

The diagnosis process is a difficult one for couples to navigate as there were things I knew were autism related and things my husband denied and wrote off as typical childhood behavior. When a man's only son is diagnosed with autism, he feels things I don't understand and will never feel. When my days are almost completely consumed with caring for a child that needs constant attention, I often have nothing left to give to my husband. It's not right, it's not fair, and I'm aware of it. But there isn't always anything I can do.

There are different theories in today's world about putting marriage first or your children first. I don't want to get involved on what I believe is right or wrong in this situation. However, I will say, to make the progress we made and to help our son in the way he needs it, the children have had to come first.

As time has gone on, we have learned how to make sure we are there for each other on top of being there for our children. It's something that every marriage has to work on, but even more so in the case of being parents to an autistic child. For me, one of the greatest sources of inspiration and enlightenment on really difficult days is knowing that my husband is the only other person that can even come close to feeling what I feel. Although we both process and handle it in different ways, there is not a single person in this outside world that knows what we are going through. WE is the keyword in this situation.

For several years, studies were going around about divorce rates as high as 80 percent for parents of autistic children. That has since been dismissed and it has been recognized that although very stressful for both parents and the marriage itself, the divorce rates are essentially standard among parents of children on the spectrum.

I would be sugarcoating if I said that this has been easy on our marriage, yet I won't go as far as to say terrible or difficult. The word I like to use is that it has been *work*. We have had to settle into what our roles are, adjust to what we can expect from each other, and recognize that we are not alone in this journey. We have no choice but to rely on each other.

OUR FAMILY

We found out I was pregnant with my daughter just a few months before my son's second birthday. She was planned. It was exactly what we wanted at the exact time. We knew our son had some quirks but it wasn't until late in my second pregnancy that things started getting out of hand. They were certainly interfering with everyday life at that point.

To this day I'm beyond grateful that we chose to expand our family at the time that we did. Had I known the road we were headed down with my son, I may have thought differently about having more children. Yet to this day, it is his sister that has pushed him the furthest, made him accomplish things we never thought he could, and truly taught him how to handle other people.

In the beginning things were terrible. I couldn't possibly be who I needed to be for a newborn and an autistic two-and-a-half-year-old. He was needy and fragile and she was colicky. There were many nights when one or the other was screaming for me while I took care of their sibling. I knew things had to get better because they didn't feel as though they could get any worse.

Eventually my son started to warm up to the idea that the baby wasn't going anywhere. The process was slow. I remember crying to the occupational therapist. I told her I've never been so happy and so sad at the same time. I was head over heels in love with my newborn daughter but at the same time she was causing my son so much distress just simply by being a baby.

I thought I set him way back and that it would take us months or years to return to where we had reached. I'll never forget the day that I was sitting on the foam mat in the OT gym with my son and our amazing OT said to me, "This is the best possible thing that could have happened to him." She was spot-on; it just took me a while to figure it out.

As the years progressed, the kids became friends. There are sibling issues like any sibling has but they love and they laugh and they teach each other things every day.

Lately I have noticed a completely different side of the dynamic that I was never aware of in the beginning.

In the beginning, I gave the baby a pacifier so she wouldn't disturb my son with her cries.

In the beginning, I kept her on a very specific schedule so that she had solid naps and he had a break from the baby at times.

In the beginning, I would lay with him to put him to bed when the baby really needed me.

Everything I did was so that myself, my husband, and my newborn daughter were making life easier on my autistic son. I was lost in it. It seemed as though I had no other choice than to make him comfortable and work everything else around that. Certainly, we tried to balance the control he had over our lives with the control we still needed to be effective parents.

This was manageable at the time. Things were fine. The baby was happy and healthy and well-adjusted. However, as she got older, something really started to bother my husband and me. She was becoming a person. She had the most adorable personality and was learning to speak. She cared for people and animals in a way that I truly admired. She knew when her brother was going to have a reaction long before I did.

She was moving out of the baby stage and becoming a little person. This transition was difficult because she wanted to do things her way, and make her own choices and decide what she needed. She was absolutely entitled to this yet it was much different than what we had experienced in the past. We could no longer let our son rule our day-to-day routine while she watched and wondered why the world revolves around her brother.

We had to adjust to make sure that she was seen as an equal part of our family and not that her brother and his issues take precedence. This has been an ongoing battle for us. Having an autistic sibling is no easy task. It's something I never gave my daughter enough credit for until recently.

There are days when she has a best friend right at her side and days when he is her worst enemy. There are no warnings as to when these days will be. She is three yet knows her brother has triggers and issues. She is very bright and has grown up fast. She talks openly in therapy about how he can't share with her and sometimes he gets mad at her.

Just recently I asked her why we go to therapy. She said, "So brother doesn't get so mad at us." She's exactly right. Behavioral therapy has changed his ability to regulate his emotions and he doesn't get nearly as mad. We started with behavioral therapy when she was only two and a half, yet in that period of time, going to therapy and observing week in and week out she is seeing that it is helping him and changing him.

This is a lot for a young child to take in. My son struggles with the fact that she is unpredictable. She is not going to have the same schedule or say the same things from day to day. Yet she too struggles with the fact that from one day to the next she's not exactly sure what will be coming her way as far as triggers and meltdowns from her brother.

It's a very difficult thing to manage. My ultimate goal as a parent is to make sure that they grow up to love and respect each other. Their relationship got off to such a rocky start I would lay awake night after night imagining them as adults who grew up to hate each other. It's my nightmare.

My son needs to know that I'm there for him always and that we have worked to change our lives and our families to better accommodate him and help him succeed.

My daughter needs to know that even though her brother is autistic and special accommodations need to be made at times, *her* feelings, needs, wants, and desires are no less important.

Having a child who couldn't tolerate going to a new park or sitting at a restaurant or a library class has changed what we do in the course of a week/year. The thing that bothers me so much is wondering if my neurotypical child will miss out on things that she would consider to be fun, just because my autistic son can't handle them.

It's a very difficult balance and one I'm sure many parents deal with on a daily basis, even with neurotypical children. The diagnosis of autism changes your family dynamics in ways that you likely didn't think were possible.

As the years go on, I think it's going to take a great deal of therapy for us all to get through this. It's very difficult for a young child to understand the complexity of autism in their sibling. The majority of *adults* in our world can't figure out autism. We can't expect a young child to figure it all out.

Here are some methods that have helped us make sure both children know and understand they are equally important:

1) **Giving each child one-on-one time when possible.**
2) **Explaining autism every single chance we get.** When an issue occurs that is related to a sensory issue or autism, it is discussed in length, regardless of the age of the child. Over time it sinks in.
3) **Teaching our autistic son how to take care of his sister.** It did not come naturally to him. He was rough and tough and didn't pay any attention to her emotional needs. He had to be taught and it has worked.
4) **Teaching our neurotypical daughter that even on the difficult days (when she is on the bad side of a meltdown) her brother loves her and doesn't want to act in the way he does.**
5) **Lots of supervision.** Sibling squabbles can be worked out fairly easily with neurotypical children. This is not the case when you throw autism into the mix. There needs to be a higher level of supervision when the kids are playing together to make sure that things go smoother and everyone is safe.
6) **Family therapy.** I've said it before and I'll say it again. WE go to therapy. It's not just my son. We don't drop him off and walk away. My daughter gets to be involved in both occupational and

behavioral therapy. She doesn't always understand *why* we are there but she knows we need to be and that it's working.

7) **Communication.** Open communication is so important on many levels, but in this instance, I'm referring to communication between myself and my husband. We are constantly trying to keep in check which child may need more from us at any given time. If my son had one of those weeks where he fought for control, my daughter may need a few hours of fishing with just Dad. As we fought to keep control of our household in our hands, she felt it. She knew we were frustrated, and so was she. There were likely games she wanted to play, things she wanted to do or see, that didn't happen because of autism.

8) **Awareness.** Making sure that not all of our decisions are made around the fact that we have an autistic child. We have two children. At times this will cause distress for our autistic son but in time he will learn that the world isn't completely about him. His sister helps him with this every day. It's a difficult lesson to learn and one we still need lots of practice. Ultimately, I (and you) want both (or all) of our children to see that they are important, respected, and loved—regardless of if they are autistic or not.

My Life

Of course, I was not the one diagnosed with autism, but I still feel as though it was a family diagnosis. My son has to deal with all of the impact but because of that my role is to lighten the burden. I work from home. I homeschool. I stay up at night when he needs it. My life has changed. I have to think three steps ahead, I have to plan things according to him almost all of the time. So much research and planning and prep work and explaining goes into even the simplest of things. It's not the life I saw. I'm not always the mom I wanted to be, but I try. The love I feel toward this child is all the motivation anyone would ever need to keep pushing along. The days can be long; the years are flying by. I've accepted the change in my life,

Me

This course in life has gone further than just impacting my life; it's actually changed who I am. I cared about certain things in life that I don't care about anymore. I worried about meaningless and frivolous things; I don't worry about them anymore. I questioned how and why people were raising their kids a certain way and I certainly don't do that anymore. Having a child on the spectrum brought my life into focus. I think any special needs parent can tell you it's all fun and games until the day you realize something is not right with your child. There is a part of you that will change.

Being goal-driven and determined, I measure my success by one accomplishment after another. Playing competitive golf my entire life, I was always ready to win the next tournament, move up a level, build a business, pay off my house etc. One goal after another—check them off the list. Having a child on the spectrum has taught me to redefine success and failure in a much different way. A success does not have to be gold-plated or Waterford crystal. In fact a success can be walking through a grocery store without headphones. A success can be wearing socks. A success can be making eye contact with a person while saying your name. These successes are not any less important or meaningful than one you can place on a mantle. This has changed me. When all is said and done, and I reach the end of my life, I will be a better person for what I have learned from my son and autism.

58

2.

EXPECTATION AND GOALS

Most great businesses start from a simple idea or one small concept and they build themselves up. Hours of work, time, effort, and money—you work your way up and grow. Sometimes you fail and fall back down that ladder and other times you fly up. It's constantly changing, always evolving, but it's a process and it is expected.

The idea of starting from scratch and working your way up is one that has been around for centuries. It's something that all Americans hope to do in their lives— to be better, accomplish more, climb those ladders. Having owned several businesses, I know this process; I know that sometimes there are complete standstills and other times things are better than you ever thought they could be.

When my son was first diagnosed, I originally imagined I was going to plan this out like a business. I would find all the deficits, all the things that didn't come naturally to him, and develop a plan to implement them. We would start at the bottom and work our way up to mastery because I know there is nothing he cannot do. We would look at social skills and sensory issues and implement them all. Choose one, mark it off our list, and get to the next one. This seemed like the best thing I could offer him—full dedication, complete mastery of all things needed to function as an independent adult someday.

Unlike the experiences I have had in business, I found that starting at the bottom and working your way up does NOT work when it comes to parenting a child on the spectrum.

Instead, if you reverse the process and start at the *top* of the ladder, you and your child will benefit in a much different way. I learned this concept from my son's early occupational therapy sessions and applied it to our lives as we acclimated to this world. The basic concept is that you start at the highest level of what you want your child to accomplish, work your way back down until something is accomplished, and then use that as your starting point to work your way back up.

For example, when we first started occupational therapy, my then two-year-old son was terrified of crawling through a fabric tunnel. The fabric bothered him. It was somewhat dark in there, it was all unknown, and he couldn't do it. So, crawling through the tunnel became the top of the expectations. Then we backed it down a step to see if we could get him to crawl partially through the tunnel. When that didn't work, we went back down another step to see if he could stick just his head in and then pop back out. When that failed miserably, we tried to have him put just one foot in while he sat outside the tunnel.

This worked.

Now we had our starting point to work back up. Today if you ask him to crawl through one of these things he would laugh and say of course he can. It just took time and work. By starting at the top and working our way down we found his highest level of tolerance and then we worked our way up from there.

So, why is this important? What would have happened had we started at the bottom?

Knowing my child, and knowing this situation, he never would have even put his foot in. He would have chosen not to go near the tunnel because it was too great of an unknown. By putting these higher demands on him and then backing it down we eventually reached a level that in his mind he thought, *Well that's not so bad compared to having to crawl through the whole thing.* Putting the foot in the tunnel may seem insignificant but it's exactly what led him to eventually being able to crawl through this tunnel with ease. He was nervous about the texture/fabric of the tunnel. Had we started at the bottom and just asked him to walk over and touch the tunnel he would have never done it. By simply reversing the ladder and starting at the top he considered all things and realized sticking one foot in was not a big deal. When he did that, he realized the fabric of the tunnel was fine. It took a month or so but eventually he navigated the tunnel with ease.

I will never be able to fully gauge the way this condition affects my son internally. I have been trained to see all the outwardly signs of distress but truly what it feels like to be him I will never know. As he's grown and been able to communicate more, I learn things every day. Since I'm not him and I can't gauge how things make him feel, why should I decide what he can and can't handle. This system has allowed both my son and our family to realize and accept what he can handle.

The tunnel may seem insignificant but it's the groundwork that we have laid that has helped with potty training and sports and it will help with future driving and college and a career. This system has surprised us numerous times. We took him to Disney World, knowing that we may have to leave at any time because of crowds and noise, only to see him ride a roller coaster and clap as a parade went by. We didn't know this would happen, but by starting at the top we *allowed it to happen* and we all have these memories to cherish forever.

A conscious effort needs to be made not to be prisoners in your own home. There will be public meltdowns and outbursts. You will walk into restaurants and have to walk out before you even get to order. You will go into a shoe store and then have to order them online. Your child will fight you, not because they want to, because they can't help it. It's a difficult, exhausting, and grueling road, but this system has done wonders for our family.

It scares to me to think of what could have happened had I decided to "protect" and "shelter" my son from all that he couldn't handle, making these decisions for him that only he can make. When I assume a birthday party or a wedding will be more than he can take, I limit his ability to reach the top of the ladder. Best-selling author, autism advocate, and animal science professor, Dr. Temple Grandin, has always been a favorite resource of mine when I need some guidance as a parent to a child with

ASD. She is brilliant and very gifted when it comes to communicating what autism is to people that don't have autism. Even though autism is a huge part of my world, I still don't have it. I still need help in figuring out what is right and what is wrong.

Probably Dr. Grandin's most helpful advice to date was released in her book *The Loving Push*. This book explains how pushing your child outside of their comfort zone to a level that is still within reason (i.e., not a meltdown) is the best way to accomplish milestones and goals.

A few inspiring quotes by Dr. Temple Grandin that resonated with me as a parent, include:

> The most important thing people did for me was to expose me to new things.

> There needs to be a lot more emphasis on what a child can do instead of what he cannot do.

> You need to stretch kids with autism slightly outside their comfort zones, but never have surprises.

> —Dr. Temple Grandin

I think the balance between push and trust is a difficult one that we monitor daily. So if pushing these children to the next level is the best thing for them, why don't all parents do this?

It is EXHAUSTING.

To be met with opposition constantly, to know that you are three seconds and two words away from an utter meltdown, is time-consuming, stressful, and taxing. It is not an easy mission for a sleep-deprived, overwhelmed, most likely financially stressed (that OT is expensive) parent. To wake up in the morning and decide to make progress is your only choice, but it is not an easy one to make.

So how does this reverse ladder system help us acclimate to our new world?

When I talk about letting everything change, because it will anyway, I use this ladder to help. I attempted our life as if we had a neurotypical child and then I adjusted from there. I worry about parents who get this diagnosis and are so lost they feel as though they need to start from scratch. You don't and you shouldn't. You need to find what rung of the ladder your child is on and then work your way up from there. The way up is the difficult part but why start at the bottom if you don't need to. I think the actual diagnosis of autism is so overwhelming for most families that plenty of things slip through the cracks and many of the positives are not focused on.

My son was terrified of the beach. If you went to put him down in the sand he would scream and climb up your body. He was young, couldn't tell me what or why the beach bothered him in this way, so we avoided it. Living in South Florida at the time it was upsetting to me. We drove past the beach constantly and I even had done his nursery in a surf theme. I would look at the hand-painted surfboard sign on the wall in his room and think, *How did this happen?* His father and I love the beach and the water so much that we enjoy traveling to see new beaches. And now we have a kid that was born HATING the beach.

When we started OT I was told it was fairly common among children with sensory issues. I told the therapist that although it may seem trivial, it is something that we want to work on. We again started high and worked our way back down. We went to the beach again to see if we could find out what exactly it is that gets to him. We discovered he loves the water and he will tolerate sitting on a towel at the beach. He just couldn't move from the towel to the water, or stand in the water himself, because of the sand. In the following months we worked on touching sand in OT and he loved it. Touching sand with his hands was not the problem. It was his feet. It took tons of role-play, lots of sensory integration, and thousands of dollars in therapy over nine months, but one Sunday morning we decided to give the beach another shot.

It started shaky. I knew he was still in the realm of being outside his comfort zone but not to meltdown level. I carried him to the water because I knew that would bring the anxiety down. I started running from a foot or two of water to the shore stating that the waves were chasing me. He was three.

"OK, I'll try now," he said.

Today we call him the sand monster when we go to the beach. This kid gets sand in places I didn't know was possible. He rolls in the sand and digs holes to lay in. He builds castles and runs and plays and throws his shoes on the boardwalk because he doesn't need or want them.

I have a picture of me standing in the water next to him on that breakthrough day and it will forever be my favorite picture of us. The emotion involved is truly indescribable. When we left the beach on that very special day, a woman who was walking her dog saw my son wet and covered in sand and said, "Well somebody loves the beach." I simply told her, "It's a long story."

This story explains everything I mean about acclimating.

His initial reactions to the sand were seen by all my family and friends. I know they all thought beach trips were done. They very likely would have been had we not chosen to allow autism to change us. We all went through a period of change and then we acclimated and now we know where we stand. The most important thing is that we didn't resist this change. We simply acclimated to our new life.

HOW TO IMPLEMENT THIS LADDER THEORY IN YOUR OWN HOME

My best tip is to pick one project at a time. As mentioned earlier, the beach was a project we worked on alone. We didn't try to simultaneously introduce new foods and playdates and soccer teams. Choose something that will have a great reward for both you and the child. If there is an activity or a food or a place that you know your child will love, focus on that first.

It's also extremely important to let your child know they are climbing this ladder. I am constantly and tirelessly saying, "Wow remember when you couldn't even _____" or "This is crazy; I was just thinking about when _____ bothered you so much we couldn't have all this fun." As the parent, your greatest joy will be seeing your child accomplish these things that once seemed impossible to accomplish. I have learned that some of the children's happiest moments are not only seeing themselves conquer and complete new things but seeing how happy their family is for them.

68

3.
COMMUNICATION

> Words are singularly the most powerful force available to humanity. We can choose to use this force constructively with words of encouragement, or destructively using words of despair. Words have energy and power with the ability to help, to heal, to hinder, to hurt, to harm, to humiliate and to humble.
>
> --Yehuda Berg

We have been lucky enough to have lots of words from a very young age. Many parents of children on the spectrum wait years and years to hear their child say their first words. I imagine it is an excruciating wait. Not knowing what is going on in your child's brain can be an extremely difficult place to be.

Even though we have had words, the communication was not always effective. My son could repeat everything you told him. It only took him hearing a word once to know what that word meant and how to use it in the right context. He would rattle off facts and questions like it was nobody's business. Yet there was still something not quite there, the communication.

Every single day I was guessing what bothered him. What trigger caused the meltdown, what had I done to make his day more difficult. When he threw himself on the ground and I would say, "What's wrong? What is bothering you?" he would just yell and scream and mostly say that nothing was bothering him. I felt, regardless of his ability to speak, we weren't getting to the bottom of what was causing him such despair.

Over time I was smart enough to figure out certain things like fabrics, a change of meal times, or taking a different route when driving to a store could cause him distress. Much of this was not because he communicated it. When it came to the way autism was affecting his thoughts and his reactions, he was not able to communicate it to myself or my husband.

With the addition of behavioral therapy and lots and lots of practice we are finally getting to a point that he can say, "I'm off today because . . ." It's not *every* day but there is progress happening. It has been completely eye-opening to me. Just when you think you have your world figured out—the triggers kept to a minimum, the environment as peaceful and regulated as possible—you find out that you don't.

Recently we took my daughter's car seat and changed it from rear-facing to forward-facing. She was a little worried about the change so I talked to her (in front of my son) about how change is difficult for all of us. I told her that her brother had a very difficult time with this same transition and he is fine now and in fact likes his seat better the way it is.

I tried to get my son involved in the conversation and helping his sister. I asked him if he remembers this and if I was correct that it was hard on him. His response shocked me and actually helped me to realize that my own progress with being a mother to an autistic child still has a long way to go.

"I remember switching car seats well," he said. "It was hard but not nearly as hard as when you changed the laundry room around."

That was the first he ever spoke about the laundry room bothering him. We had a shelf in the laundry room that was not effective so I bought a new one that would better store our things. He shopped with me for it, helped me put it together, and seemed fine. I tried to remember if he seemed to struggle after we changed the laundry room but it was hard for me, because the laundry room change was more than seven months prior!

All this time he had a terrible time with the fact that we changed our laundry room and he kept it to himself. I know changes for holidays when we decorate and take decorations down affect him. I know if something in his room changes that he is upset by it. A shelf in the laundry room? I just didn't even think about it. In fact with his involvement in the process I thought he enjoyed the new shelf.

The moral of the story here is that this was actually a very good increase in communication for my son. And for that I am thankful. However, this also provided a very good realization into the fact that I am not autistic and, as much as I figure out and help him and work on things, I will never know what goes on inside his brain. For me it's like climbing a ladder that has no top rung.

Each day I learn more. I won't ever reach the top of the ladder but it's one that I don't mind climbing. It helps him as I move up the ladder. And as he learns to communicate better, we can deal with things before they bother him as opposed to after. That will be a very big day for all of us.

4.

ELIMINATING COMPARISONS

The final part of acclimation is the key ingredient to your continued mental health. I use a simple method that I was taught as a kid before crossing a street—Stop, Look, and Listen. This phrase has helped me to cross many a busy street in my life—especially the twelve-lane highway I'm currently trying to navigate, also known as parenting a child on the spectrum.

First, a little backstory as to how I came up with this method and how it has changed my mindset.

It was a typical Saturday afternoon out in our town. Since the whole babysitter thing doesn't work all that well in our life, and we don't live near family, we try to go to a happy hour now and then. My husband and I have a beer and an appetizer and we order the kids a meal. Seems simple. It's not.

Understandably, sitting in a crowded loud restaurant would be difficult for an autistic child but this battle starts well before that. My husband and I play Rock, Paper, Scissors to choose who has to tell him that we are going out that day. We both know that if the routine is changed there will be consequences for all of us.

We have tried telling our son about an outing days before, or the day of, or not until we leave the house, but there are no great solutions. If we tell him too soon and then the schedule changes again, we pay for it twice.

Again, there's just no perfect solution, aside from not leaving the house at all (which is not an option for us).

Whoever draws the short stick gets to tell him that we will be going out that afternoon. He, of course, doesn't handle it well, says he's not going, falls to the floor, all the usual things. We look at each other and debate as to if this is worth it and we almost always decide that it is. Roughly 99.9 percent of the time we decide it *is* worth pushing through our son's comfort zone (for things we know he will enjoy) and try to use our time together as a family effectively. We go to places that we know are nearly empty. We go at such times that people have trouble figuring out if we are eating a late lunch, an early dinner, or what we are even doing at the restaurant then. We sit outside when we can. We bring headphones and games for distraction. We go to familiar places and if it is unfamiliar, we look at pictures before we go. We spend a good hour of our day dealing with just being able to leave the house to go and do something like this and the entire outing rarely lasts more than an hour.

Hours of work for an hour of "normalcy." Doesn't seem worth it, but for our sanity it is. We have all become so accustomed to his reactions to our plans that we are just able to deal with it when it comes. If we did not push through and see his joy with handling an experience or an event I think we all would be in a very different mental place.

The crazy part about this is when all is said and done, he has fun. It's a good time for our family and we enjoy our time. It's some of the best memories that we have. It's just work, constant work. On one of these adventures a few years back, while trying to simultaneously eat a nacho, nurse a baby, distract a toddler with autism, have a conversation with my husband, and convince myself I was having a great time, I started looking at other families around the restaurant. I always observe people and dynamics but this day was different. I truly started feeling sorry for myself, for my son, and our family.

I looked at every table and thought:

- Did they dread telling their child they were going out that day, or did that thought not even cross their mind?

- Did they have to plan ahead where they went and what time, or do they just get in the car and go?

- Did they have to battle about which shoes and socks felt right or clothes that were not itchy but still nice enough to wear in a restaurant, or do they just put clothes out and their child puts them on?

- Did they have to bring a calm down kit or headphones or sometimes just walk out if the conditions (lighting/sound/breading on the chicken fingers) were not just perfect?

- Did they have to call ahead of time to make sure their chicken fingers were crunchy but not spicy? Thin and not thick?

- Did they have to adjust the buckle on the seatbelt twelve times to make sure it is not too loose, but not too tight, and then have to keep checking to make sure said seatbelt stays on?

75

- What would it be like to just say, "Hey kids, get in the car. We are going out to eat."

I couldn't imagine what it would have been like. I don't even know how to function in a way that doesn't include forty-seven steps and mental checklists. I wouldn't know where to start. Maybe I'm not cut out for that type of carefree lifestyle, but it did have me wondering. It made me guess if they had more fun than we do, if their life was overall less stressful, what they did with their extra time that wasn't used to chase after shoes being flung at you when you try and leave the house.

All the people on this earth have a different road. I'm sure there are things they deal with in their everyday life that I don't ever want to deal with or wouldn't be cut out for. I let this questioning, this sadness, linger for a few days and then the realization hit me that it was doing me no good.

As I talked about at the beginning of the book, once you put those autism glasses on that is it. My brain does not know how to function as a "normal" mom anymore. I have to see and think and be three steps ahead at all times. It is my only choice and clearly I AM cut out for it. Comparing to other families and wondering what their reality is was getting me nowhere.

That's when it hit me. *Stop, Look, and Listen.*

STOP: Stop comparing.
LOOK: Look at how far you have come.
LISTEN: Listen to yourself. *This is our path.*

STOP

There is lots of talk about this in all the latest parenting magazines and scholarly articles. I recently read an Instagram post from a woman with triplets (two girls and one boy). Her boy was doing things a bit slower than the girls and right away she thought he was autistic. Sad. I don't blame this mother one bit. It's a fear that all parents have and every time you compare your child to another the thought goes through your mind that there may be something wrong with your child. So many factors go into child development the average parent can't be able to truly compare one child to another.

For this step it's important to remember to not just stop comparing one child to another, it's also imperative not to compare one family to another and one parent to another. Not only do all families function in different ways but the difference between special needs families and neurotypical families can be remotely different. I could never really get involved in the playground stay-at-home moms' talks. I'm just not good at them and I would second-guess my child for weeks to come. He was not able to walk on the sand at the park (just like the beach, he hated sand, and it was too unpredictable when he put his foot down) yet he was spelling things on the swing. Mothers would ask me questions about him and he would answer for himself. He once walked into therapy at two and a half years old and said, "You mind signing me in, Mom?" He proceeded to spell his name for me as if I didn't know. There were other parents in the waiting room with children who couldn't say "Mama" at the same age. I'm sure they compared their child. I'm sure it hurt and I almost wanted to say, "Yes, I know that was amazing, but . . ." The same goes for watching another mother with her child. She may seem harder/softer/more direct/more scattered/whatever it may be because it works for *her child*, not yours.

One thing that can help a lot to "STOP" is to quit people watching so much. It's hard. I like it; I always have. I like knowing all that is going on around me at all times, but I had to stop paying such close attention to other families, parents, children, and their dynamic. It was too different than what we dealt with. Now when I see a child happily hand flapping running across a park I do feel a certain sense of closeness to the mother of that child, a bond that only certain people *get*.

LOOK

I don't care who you are or who your child is, you have made some level of progress. If your progress is just the fact that you are reading this book to get a better level of understanding, you have made progress. Progress is defined as a forward movement toward a destination. I'm sure we all have a different destination in mind but each day we are making progress. Sometimes progress looks like a good school day, or wearing shoes, or licking an apple, but you need to constantly remind yourself of how far you have come.

One way that has helped me remember our progress is blogging. When we first found out about sensory processing disorder, I started a blog to educate family and friends and I used it as an outlet for myself. I love that I have these blog posts to go back to and read and reminisce about how far we have come. Start a journal, write about the really bad days. It's amazing therapy. Keep writing and a year from now open that journal back to the beginning and see how far you have come.

Over time I have noticed that people that don't see us for a while are amazed at how far my son has come—to the point that I question myself and think, *Wow, I guess it was that bad.* These writings have helped me to look back and realize what I missed being caught up in the day-to-day adventures and happenings.

LISTEN

There will be a day when your child walks into a building and the lighting is just "off." The lighting is off and it throws them off. You don't know if it's too bright or too dark but you know you have just lost them. They will be mid-meltdown, and while trying to help them and yourself, you will catch the glares of quite a few people. It's going to happen. None of us are immune. When this happens, I simply remind myself, *This is our path.* In the next section of the book when we talk about amplitude, I will get more into this and how to use it to help you. The main focus is to get the mindset that this is your path. The meltdown is happening for a reason. It might be a learning moment for your child, for yourself, or (and this one has been a huge realization for me) it might be for an onlooker. The person staring might have had a nail in their tire yesterday and thought their world was coming to an end. When they witness what your day to day is, it may change them. You will likely never know this but it is a HUGE source of power when it comes to these difficult moments in parenting a child on the autistic spectrum.

The other part is to listen to those around you. No, not the ones who try to tell you how to parent your child, nor the ones who don't believe in autism. It's also not the ones who say that your kid needs some discipline or it's just the terrible twos. Listen to the ones that say, "Wow, I give you a lot of credit." Or the one that says "You have come so far." I shrugged it off for too many years and now I'm here to LISTEN. If another mom wants to tell me that they see a positive change in my child, I'm going to listen. I'm going to take that information and soak it in and realize that these are the positive affirmations I need to get me through the rough days.

The Stop, Look, and Listen system is very easy to follow and it's something you can start working on tomorrow. The changes will happen immediately for your mindset. What I have noticed about my life and the life of my child since doing this is that there is less stress. I don't feel as pressured to compete and compare to other families. Living our life, our story without distraction or pressure from outside influences is the ultimate goal.

KEY REMINDERS
FROM THE ACCLIMATION PROCESS

- Find what rung of the ladder your child is on and then work your way up from there.

- A conscious effort needs to be made not to be prisoners in your own home.

- Comparing yourself to other families and wondering what their reality is will get you nowhere. Not only do all families function in different ways, but the difference between special needs families and neurotypical families can be remotely different.

- You have made some level of progress. Even the fact that you are reading this book to get a better level of understanding is progress.

- Stop, Look, and Listen.

THIRD STEP

AMPLITUDE

(THE WHY, THE DIFFERENCES BETWEEN THE HIGHS AND LOWS, AND HOW TO USE THESE TO PROPEL YOU INTO THE FUTURE)

1.

FUEL FOR THE BAD DAYS

You have reached my favorite part of this book. We already discussed and laid out how to approve of your new life, approve of autism, approve of your child and the future that you all have together. We have covered how to acclimate to this life, steps to take to lessen the burden (especially the mental burden), how to not only survive but to prosper and grow together as well. These two steps are very powerful and they will without a doubt change the way you and your family function. The part that is missing is the why. *Why did this happen to me, why does nobody understand this like I do, and why couldn't we just be normal?*

Through years of thinking and studying and writing and analyzing, I fully believe that I have embraced the why. Not just for parenting a child on the spectrum but for any special needs parenting.

The definition of amplitude that we are using deals with electricity. Amplitude is the maximum deviation of an alternating current from its average value. Essentially, how far we can travel from the average in both a positive and negative way. There are thousands of stories that can describe this theory of amplitude but I'll offer a few that will help you understand the impact and how you can use this as fuel in your daily lives.

My son was just two years old. He had shown some quirky behaviors but at the time it was still too hard to distinguish if it was sensory or toddler. While playing in the yard with him I noticed his shoes seemed small all of a sudden. I took a look and determined that he most definitely needed a new pair of sneakers. With nothing else really going on that day I loaded him up in the car and drove the fifteen minutes to the local Shoe Carnival.

He knew we were getting new shoes; we talked about it. He was fine with the idea. He asked if he could get blue and I was more than cool with that. We walked into the store and he was quiet and polite and stayed right by my side as he always did. I grabbed a pair of shoes off the shelf in the next size up, opened the box, and my world that I was living in disappeared.

The world of "basic toddler life." The world without therapy appointments and charts and signs and social cues and worry upon worry upon worry. It was gone. He took one look at the new shoes and he lost it. He couldn't handle that they were not the same as what he had on; he couldn't tolerate that there was going to be something new on his feet when he had just barely learned to accept the ones he had. He was inconsolable and all I had done was open the shoe box. He ran through the store, up and down the aisles, completely unreachable. One store employee asked me if I needed help and I remember saying, "I'm not even sure what I need." Luckily there were not very many people in the store at the time, although even if there were, I'm not sure I saw them.

I chased my son right out the door of the store. The boy that had never been more than three feet from me his entire life. I never thought he would run; I had never even seen him react like this. Sure, he was picky about socks and shoes and how they were put on and I knew these were all little red flags but this was extreme. This was new, it was severe, and unfortunately it was the first of many. When we got back in the car, he was hysterical. I remember working on making sure he breathed in and out and tried to get him to relax. It was nearly impossible. When I felt like he was calm enough, I buckled up and drove home.

We didn't talk much on that ride. I simply told him everything would be fine and we would work this out. A few minutes before we got home, he regained his composure and said something that will forever resonate in my mind. He said, "I'm sorry I don't mean to act like that." He was two.

At two years old he told me that there was something not right. For him to tell me that something was just not right and he doesn't want to act like that was the information I needed to call the doctor and get him into OT and start our journey. Of course, when he said this to me—his tiny bare feet, his blond hair, and baby blue eyes—I looked in my rearview mirror and the waterworks started. It was one of the biggest moments of both of our lives and it was all about a pair of shoes.

After six or eight months of occupational therapy, when he needed another new pair of shoes, I confided to the therapist that I was scared to take him into a shoe store. She understood completely and agreed. She told me to order a few pairs of shoes and bring them to therapy so we could work on it together. We worked on it, we prepped him and taught him and talked him through it and at the end of the session he was wearing his new shoes.

For the rest of my life, when I see my son put a pair of shoes on, I will experience a level of joy that parents of neurotypical children cannot comprehend. This is our why. This is our bonus and we have earned it. The amplitude, the difference between the terrible moments and the moments that we can't even believe are real-life, is extreme.

These extremes happen daily. There is a meltdown in the morning and that night they try their first karate class. Karate class, new shoes, a piece of cheese—these are not things that all parents get to enjoy in this way.

You do. That is a gift.

If you do not recognize these gifts and use them to fuel you through the difficult times, you will be missing out on the entire "why" behind parenting a child on the autistic spectrum.

The question then becomes HOW to use this as your fuel. How do you not lose your cool, and get depressed and hide in your home before you even have the chance to see the opposite end of this crazy spectrum. One of the best activities to help you realize the fuel is to choose your top three worst meltdowns or aversions. We all have had them; the public ones are messy, but you and I know the ones at home can be just as bad.

Take those three moments and ask yourself what caused them. Most of the time you can figure out a trigger—why your child was off that day, why they were affected in the way they were. If you think about this it won't be hard for you to come up with something. Now take that same trigger and think about how it affects your child today. Is it the same? Are they able to tolerate it? Would their reaction be the same as it once was?

In some cases, it may be but from what I have found is that over time the worst of the worst do gradually improve. You need to find out what these three greatest improvements have been. Find your biggest differences between the lowest of the lows and the highest of the highs.

The very next time your child struggles (something simple like the breading on the nuggets at Chick-fil-A), remember this.

It's so that when they call you someday and say they just stopped and got themselves lunch at Chick-fil-A you can smile. You will think back to this day and you will remember how frustrated you were. You will remember how difficult it was to keep your cool and to relax and realize it's just a chicken nugget. You will think back to how all you were doing was trying to give them that "normal" childhood that you so badly felt they deserved. Well, it worked; it was worth it.

Know this ahead of time. Know that the gift you were given being the parent of a special needs child is that the highs are going to be the highest of the highs. You are strong, your child is stronger. Use these difficult moments, the days that never end, the sleepless nights. Use them for fuel. Truthfully, you are going to *need* this fuel to power you through. I've come a long way in my personal development since my son was born and I have a long way to go. I have changed my mindset over and over again and I have most certainly had those days where I wholeheartedly believed I didn't have what it takes to be the mother of a child with ASD.

Each time I had these thoughts, something would bring me back to the reality that I am cut out for this position. *That* is amplitude.

2.

THEY JUST DON'T GET IT

Now that we have discussed the idea and concept behind amplitude, we come to what in my opinion is the hardest and most difficult step of this entire process. This is a step that has taken me a long time to master. It has caused me more setbacks and heartaches than any other part of the journey. That being said, and while sticking with the theme of amplitude and highs and lows, mastering this step has been the greatest advancement in my personal development since I started on this journey. This is the thing that made me feel like an adult (even though I technically was one) almost overnight. It's put ME back in control of my life and how I feel and what our future is going to look like.

When my son was younger, his grandparents were visiting and he took a fall in the driveway. It was a pretty nasty fall and he had two scraped knees. Nothing requiring an ER visit but painful. This was the first time he had scraped a knee in this way. He was right around two and a half years old. He wanted me and only me to help him and I was fine with that. The pain wasn't the problem. I quickly learned that he couldn't handle the fact that his skin had changed. He was screaming at his knees to heal. He was asking us exactly how many minutes it would be until his knees looked like they should. He could not move on. It took hours.

I held him, I talked him down, we tried to distract and nothing worked. My husband asked his parents to just give us space and let us try and calm him. Eventually (by the grace of God) I had the thought that if he couldn't *see* it, he might feel better. Ninety-seven degrees in South Florida at the time and I told him we had to put sweatpants on. The SECOND they were on he stopped crying, calmed down, ran outside and asked his grandparents if they were ready to play again. My father-in-law came inside and told my husband and me, "That was a little extreme for a scraped knee."

I remember explaining (with the support of my husband) that this was sensory related. Our son's system doesn't even know how to process pain, let alone a change in his skin. I tried to explain why putting pants on would help him because he could take a mental break from the idea and use the skills he has to help calm him down. We have learned so much since then that we now know if he falls and gets hurt, he wants to take a shower right away. He gets so much anxiety about how the water will hurt the cut at the end of the day when he showers that it will ruin his entire day. Now if he falls, he's pretty tough. He takes a quick shower, puts on clothing that covers the area, and goes about his day like nothing happened. The extreme reaction is not and never has been a choice.

While explaining this to my father-in-law I felt like he wasn't understanding. I kept trying to talk about how his system is just different than ours and how we are still in the process of figuring out all that we need to know. I went on a rant about what we had learned at OT and why we do certain things the way we do. He was politely listening to me and nodding his head but I know he thought I was nuts. I suspect he thought I was babying this boy. That when a kid falls you tell them they are fine and you move on with your day. Truly there is nothing I want more than for this to be the case, but it's not our path.

For days I tortured my husband telling him that I needed to find some way to help his father understand that this wasn't my parenting, that it was sensory related. I started finding articles, asking my husband if I should share this with his family, and we both agreed we would try and educate in small amounts. Nobody likes a boatload of information coming at them. Through the years we have tried to give out bits of information to all of our family to help them better understand our son, our lifestyle choices, our plans for the future etc. To back up our often-doubted parenting skills. I always took the looks and the questions as a personal attack on my parenting when in reality it was probably just a lack of understanding. We thought education would help.

There was a statement that my husband and I were saying to each other almost daily. It was something that would come up at least once in a situation throughout the day, whether it be in response to family or friends or someone in a store. We always said, "They just don't get it."

They just don't get it.

It was said depressingly, almost in a defeated tone, like it wasn't even worth explaining anymore. It made us feel different and alone and sometimes outcast—until we learned how to channel this thought in the correct way for our mental health and the benefit of our children.

We edited this thought/statement to include. . .

They just don't get it, **and they never will**.

The revised statement seems even more harsh, doesn't it? It's more permanent with no sign of hope. The truth is it has changed our lives. It releases all of those around us of having to understand. The truth is, they never will. Unless you live in this house, unless this is your child, unless you have been firsthand to witness these super lows and these crazy highs, you WILL NOT get it. So why do we expect people to?

Mostly because it's scary and lonely when you first find out your child needs help. You want your family and friends and your world to be supportive and with you. They will be with you, some will support you, but they won't *get it*. When you have a colicky newborn and your autistic three-year-old can't tolerate noise, nobody will get it. When you walk into bowling alleys and restaurants and walk right out because the noise or the lighting is not ideal. When you choose to homeschool because you know it's the right choice for your child and your family. When you limit his schedule and allow him lots of time at home. When you take two months to try and introduce a new food instead of just handing it to your child. When you plan and prep and research and coordinate every single part of a vacation or outing out of the house and it still goes wrong. Nobody will get it.

They never will because it's not their journey, it's not their path. Letting go of the expectation that others will understand what our day to day is like has been truly magical. My husband and I both have said that we feel as though we have grown as humans faster than we thought possible. I don't go on rants about sensory exposure or vestibular input. I skip conversations regarding new theories around causes, treatments, and developments. It's not worth my time. My time is best spent on helping my child.

It helps that people know your child is autistic but your time must be spent on helping your child develop and prosper in this world. You cannot dedicate your life to helping others understand your child. It just doesn't work like that when you look at the long-term goals that need to be accomplished. There is not enough time or information to get outsiders to understand this diagnosis in the same way you do.

Your child, however, does get it. You don't need to explain autism to them in this way. They know the feelings. They know what it's like, even more than you do. This makes shifting your energy to your child a very easy transition.

There are plenty of people in our lives that ask questions about autism and I'm happy to answer. I just spend a lot less time trying to ensure understanding. It does not matter if they know what our day to day looks like; it matters that I'm helping my child learn how to navigate this world as an autistic person.

The letting go of the expectation has given my husband and me so much more power. When we say no or yes to things, we simply say yes or no. We don't care what anyone else thinks of these decisions because they are made with our son's best interest in place. We also don't explain these decisions to anyone anymore. Most importantly, and the hardest part of all, we don't care what anyone else thinks because . . . *they don't get it and they never will.*

Just as if someone has a child with food allergies or cerebral palsy or a lazy eye, I have no idea what you are going through and I never will. I choose not to comment on your parenting because I'm sure you made those decisions with your child's best interest in mind.

Once while at an occupational therapy appointment with my son, I started talking to another mother. Our appointment times coincided for a few weeks in a row so we started with some small talk about our children's ages etc. She started speaking about why she was there and the issues her daughter struggled with. Her daughter was not autistic and instead had issues with seizures and tumors. A very different life than I know. Her stories were fascinating, her battles sounded difficult, her future seemed a bit uncertain and I was genuinely interested in what she had to say. I listened to the way she spoke about all that she dealt with and realized she was struggling. I tried to offer support and encouragement and pick out a few of the brighter things that she had said.

The conversation eventually turned to why I was there. I explained that my son was autistic. Now before I got a chance to explain anything at all she said, "Ha. My friends have autistic kids. I *wish* my kid was autistic." I didn't know what to say. My first thought was to defend my son's struggles, my battles with trying to help him, this journey that we are on. I thought about trying to explain how he wouldn't eat, get dressed, sleep or communicate. Then I remembered my statement, my new mindset: *They just don't get it and they never will.*

I would like to say that she didn't mean anything by her comment but I think she did. I think to her autism looks easy. I can't say that my life is harder than hers. I can't say that her life is harder than mine. We are each on our journeys for a reason.

What she said wasn't right to say to another special needs mom. The fact that she wished autism on her child helped me realize even more that no amount of explaining could be done to get her to understand. She never would. I chose to let it be. I made a broad statement about how I'm sure her days are very difficult.

I'm proud of my son that he can handle himself so well in day-to-day life that people question, is he autistic? Or as in the case above, assume that autism is easy. My favorite question is when people say, "Are you sure he is even autistic?"

Yes, I'm 100 percent certain that he is autistic. I never question it. Even on the good days I know there are still signs and I've learned to embrace these signs and autism itself.

Meltdowns often happen for us behind closed doors. As my son gets older, he handles things overall much better but at home he does have meltdowns. With family or friends over this is very rare. When I describe a meltdown of his to our family and friends, they can be very skeptical as to how bad it was. "Did it last hours? Did he actually get violent? He always seems fine." This has been difficult for me. I feel as though people think I'm complaining or looking for attention, when it's not at all the case. My sister-in-law once witnessed a full-blown meltdown. She didn't need to say anything to me; she looked at me and I knew she knows I've never exaggerated a bit of this.

If you have made it this far in this book, you owe it to yourself to start accepting the fact that they don't get it and they never will. It will take a tremendous amount of stress out of your life. It will add back in the normalcy that I know you so desperately need. When you have the desire to start trying to defend and explain, just stop yourself. Take that motivation, the drive, and turn it toward helping your child. Read about new developments. Come up with new strategies. Practice a social skill with them. Anything but letting others' thoughts feelings, and actions run your life.

> No one saves us but ourselves. No one can and no one may. We ourselves must walk the path.
>
> —Buddha

There is so much about autism that can't be controlled and yet our children crave control and order in their lives.

You cannot control how another person views you, how they understand autism, or if they accept the diagnosis or your strategies. All that you can control is your mindset. Allowing yourself to be thrown off by the fact that those around you do not get it leads to only poor outcomes for you or your child.

3.

EMPATHY AND PEOPLE

> I know it might sound weird, but empathy is one of the
> greatest creators of energy. It's counterintuitive because it's
> selfless.
>
> —Angela Ahrendts

At the time of diagnosis, I was told that my son would struggle with empathy. Autism can severely affect a person's ability to relate to and understand other humans. I already saw signs of this. When we said the classic, "How would you like it if someone did that to you?" he would just say, "I wouldn't care." This would infuriate my husband and me, because he really meant it.

He wasn't just saying he wouldn't care; he actually *meant* he wouldn't care.

When we would explain that his sister's feelings could get hurt by his actions or words, he would not understand. He wasn't trying to be difficult or disobey. He looked at us with a blank look like we didn't know what we were saying.

This was difficult on me as a parent because my ultimate goal is to raise good humans—people who care about other people, and our earth, animals, and causes. It felt like this was going to be a challenge when it came to my son. I started thinking about all the things he couldn't do in the past and all the things he is now capable of.

I remembered a time when he couldn't look anyone in the eye or say hello or even wave. How about when he refused to wear clothing or shoes, or even eat somedays. All of these things had to be worked toward, taught, practiced, and eventually achieved. Why couldn't we take the same approach with empathy?

This is exactly what we did.

I started looking for ways to expose my son to causes, people that needed help, people that were different (just like he is different). I knew that I would need outside sources to help teach him these things. We found a local organization where kids can come in and pack bags of food for other children in the community who are hungry on weekends. The system they use is very methodical. It's an assembly line of placing items in bags and then putting them in a container at the end.

Eventually my son learned all of the steps involved and then wanted to learn about restocking, deliveries, and other processes that took place. He wanted to be as involved as he could with this organization. At the time, his growing interest was not because of the mission (to feed hungry children); it was about the system.

Each time we left I would say: "You did such a great job today feeding hungry children." "We are so lucky to not be hungry." "I know these kids are thankful to have you in their lives because of all of your hard work." I would bring the people element back into the picture for my son. He saw food going in bags and I subtly but methodically reminded him that real people, real children consume this food. We went every week, for a month, three months, six months, nine months. . . and then the breakthrough started happening.

He was finishing his lunch one day and there was a bit of a granola bar left on his plate. He looked at his food, looked at me, and said, "Is there any possible way not to waste this? Any possible way to give it to one of the hungry children?" Boom. Lightbulb went off. We were moving towards empathy. *I can't finish my food but there is another hungry human that potentially could.*

This was almost two years ago now and the increase in his understanding of people and people that need help has dramatically changed.

This year he was given money that he could put toward a charitable use. He told us that he wanted to buy some toys for his therapist to use for the other children during play therapy. His exact words were: "I would really like to help someone that has helped me."

Statements like this absolutely change everything I've ever thought I've known about autism. It is now fully my belief that autistic people can learn to be empathetic—just as they can learn to communicate and socialize and handle the beach or restaurants. There will be things that my son will enjoy more than others but his life will be fuller because of the introduction of these things that autism would otherwise push out.

To bring it back to amplitude. . .

When you have spent your life volunteering and donating and caring for people of all types, it can be difficult to hear that your child cannot understand empathy. Every parent would be proud of a child who volunteers their time, puts in effort, works to help someone less fortunate. Now, take the parent who was told their child can't "feel" toward other people in this way. Watch that parent's face when their child says they want to use their birthday money to buy food for hungry people or bring some dog toys to the shelter or buy a toy for a foster child. This is the amplitude. The difference between what it was supposed to be, and what it is, is so great that you cannot even describe the feeling.

KEY REMINDERS
FROM THE AMPLITUDE PROCESS

- The difference between the highs and lows are the why that all special needs parents need to focus on.

- They just don't get it, and they never will.

- Letting go of the expectation that others will understand what our day to day is like is truly magical.

- Your time is best spent on helping your child.

- You cannot dedicate your life to helping others understand your child.

Afterword

Remembering Your Role

WHEN YOUR CHILD is born, you see nothing but the future. You don't even remember a time when you didn't have them in your arms. You can't think about what you did to keep yourself entertained and you can't even comprehend what made life special before you met them. Your days are filled with hopes and dreams and thoughts of what this child can do with their lives and for our world. They have a completely clean slate in front of them and your job, your role, your purpose in life is to help them. There are millions of ways to help them, and you will make lots of mistakes along the way, but the only thing that matters is that you help them.

As your child grows and the signs of autism emerge, you will become tired. Your role of "helping" them will take on an entirely different meaning. You will be tired of medical bills, insurance, nutrition problems, sleep issues, meltdowns, and sensory processing struggles. You will be tired. This level of exhaustion will wear you down. No parent is immune from this and it's OK to admit.

My son has almost never slept through a night in his life. These parents that say their babies sleep through the night when they are four months old are people that I honestly can't even relate to. There is no simple way to say it, I get very worn down. When this first started happening, I felt as though it was something wrong with me. Now (I'm older) I know I'm not the only one that feels this way.

Some people deal with the speech and communication issues. We are on the opposite end of the spectrum and deal with high IQ and constant (I mean, not stopping to even breathe) questioning. The questioning lasts all day and continues into the night. Some questions come up at 2 a.m. Questions come up while I try to use the bathroom. Questions come up midway through brushing teeth. They are endless. There is no way to have conversations without my son being involved. You can't put the news on because he will listen to it, memorize it, and then repeat/harp over all things that were said for days, if not weeks.

This is not like having "young kids." This is something entirely different.

With the constant demands, the lack of interaction with the outside world, and the disappearance of any kind of sleep, there is no possible way to stay at 100 percent. The very idea of self-care is laughable at times. I'm supposed to be taking time for myself but I just don't know when that time is. I don't even know what I would want to do. Sleep might be nice but I'm not sure I want to even show my body what sleep is in case it likes it.

Over time what I have found was that the more run down I got the less I liked myself as a mom. I started feeling like my relationship with my son was changing. Of course, it had to change a little as I went from being his mom to his caregiver, his teacher, his push, his pull, his trust, his fall back, his security blanket, his psychologist, his therapist, his OT—and I'm not even sure this covers it all. When I'm exhausted, I focus on goals and stats and plans and progress. I don't lead with my heart as much as I should.

When I'm managing things well, I focus on my son. The person. The child that I couldn't love more if I tried. The kid who makes me laugh, smile, and cry more than any other person ever has. The one who taught me how strong I am. The one who brought tears to my eyes the day he ate a piece of cheese. He has made me experience the ups (and occasionally downs) of life like no one else ever could.

He is the same person I gave birth to, the same child he was the day before he was diagnosed with sensory processing disorder, and the same child he was the day before he was diagnosed with autism. He is a brilliant, hardworking individual that never asked for any of this and deserves a mother who leads with her heart. He deserves love and he has earned the right to be a child.

So how does this all apply to you? I'm sure you can relate to much of what I have said but there is a key takeaway.

It is very easy to forget your role as a parent of a child on the autistic spectrum. **Your role is to love them.** I'm guilty of overplanning, overprepping, overanalyzing, and missing the actual life events. I always try and stay one step ahead and be ready for something that might come up but it has made me miss things.

There are days and times when I look at a situation and I feel like I step out of the mom role and become a therapist or a psychologist. I've accepted that to help my son thrive this is something that needs to happen. The most important part is that I resume being Mom as soon as I possibly can.

You must never forget that your role is their parent.

You must never forget that your child *does* need you to guide them through these difficult things they were handed.

You must never forget that their chance at independence and freedom and happiness is most greatly impacted by you and you alone. Your instinct and your love are enough to get this job done. This is exactly why your mental health and processing of this diagnosis and the effects it will have on you is of the utmost importance, now and for the rest of your life.

ADDITIONAL RESOURCES

Through the years, I have found many groups, blogs, and Instagram accounts that have helped me in my journey. Each style of parenting will be different, and what helps me on any given day, may or may not be helpful to you. Here are a few of my favorites.

The Out of Sync Child- a book by Carol Kranowitz
https://out-of-sync-child.com/

MyLittlePoppies-a great resource for Homeschooling and teaching children. Especially children that may not learn using traditional methods.
https://my-little-poppies.com/

The OT Toolbox- loads of Occupational Therapy tips and tricks for those days when you need to be an OT
https://www.theottoolbox.com/

Organization for Autism Research- has some great pamphlets and books on a variety of topics
https://researchautism.org/

ACKNOWLEDGMENTS

To my children, the inspiration for this book, and for everything I do.

To my husband, for your support when I told you I needed to share our story.

To my Mom for paving the way as to what it means to be a Mother.

For all of the family and friends who have understood, helped, cut a bit of slack, and loved on my boy. For that, I will be forever grateful.

ABOUT THE AUTHOR

Britt Olizarowicz is a former golf professional turned work at home Mother and freelancer. When her young son started showing signs of Sensory Processing Disorder and eventually Autism, Britt felt compelled to share the journey. In the early days, when her son could barely tolerate noise of any kind, he would request to drive on "Quiet Highways," hence the title for her first book. Britt is open and honest about what life is like for a parent of a child on the spectrum. Her ultimate goal is to make the life of one other parent just a little easier. Britt lives in Savannah, GA, with her husband, son, and daughter.

Made in the USA
Middletown, DE
13 April 2021

37435517R00071